CW01368780

Mis-Understanding ADHD

The complete guide for parents to alternatives to drugs

Dr Sami Timimi

AuthorHouse™
1663 Liberty Drive, Suite 200
Bloomington, IN 47403
www.authorhouse.com
Phone: 1-800-839-8640

AuthorHouse™ UK Ltd.
500 Avebury Boulevard
Central Milton Keynes, MK9 2BE
www.authorhouse.co.uk
Phone: 08001974150

© 2007 Dr Sami Timimi. All rights reserved.

No part of this book may be reproduced, stored in a retrieval system, or transmitted by any means without the written permission of the author.

First published by AuthorHouse   3/21/2007

ISBN: 978-1-4259-8829-6 (sc)

Printed in the United States of America
Bloomington, Indiana

This book is printed on acid-free paper.

Contents

Preface ix

Acknowledgements xvii

Part 1   Theoretical Perspectives   xix

Chapter 1 *Myths and facts*   1

Myth 1: Attention deficit hyperactivity disorder (ADHD) is a mental illness/psychiatric disorder that can be reliably diagnosed and occurs in similar numbers of children regardless of their cultural background. It affects between 3 and 10% percent of all children, is a lifelong disorder and leads to serious disability in the young person's ability to learn, socialise, work, and otherwise lead a normal life.   2

Myth 2: ADHD is caused by irregularities in brain chemistry and runs in families. Scientists have identified malfunctioning genes that disrupt communications between different cells in parts of the brain that are in charge of self-control and inhibition.   11

Myth 3: Stimulants such as Ritalin are a first line treatment of choice for ADHD. Stimulants are safe and effective. Drug treatment may need to be given for the rest of that person's life.   15

Myth 4: Treatment for ADHD with medication improves public health with minimum risks.   28

Myth 5: Any treatment for ADHD type behaviours that does not include medication is unlikely to be successful.   29

Chapter 2 *Making sense of the scientific evidence*   31

The Role Of Meaning: 35
Positivism: 38
Culture And Social Construction: 41
Meaning And Values: 44
The Spectre Of Eugenics: 49

Some Concluding Thoughts:	63
Chapter 3 *ADHD as a medical condition*	64
A Brief History Of ADHD:	66
Western Childhoods:	71
The Medicalisation Of Childhood:	82
A Crisis For Children?	95
ADHD And Children's Temperament:	100
Attachment To Fathers And Mothers:	100
Reframing The Problem:	102
Modern Lifestyles:	107
Changes In The Way We Parent:	110
Changes In Our Education System:	111
The Influence Of Living In A Market Economy And Consumerism:	113
Why So Many Boys?	122
The Role Of Governments:	129
Chapter 5 *Developing a multi-perspective approach*	130
The Power Of Language:	131
Science, Bias, And Globalisation:	132
Developing A Value System:	136
Part 2 **Practical Alternatives To Drugs**	145
Chapter 6 *On using this section*	147
How To Use This Section:	151
Chapter 7 *Common pitfalls*	153
Giving Up Too Quickly:	153
Becoming Hopeless Following A Setback:	154
Unrealistic Expectations:	155
Inconsistency:	157

Unresolved Parental Relationship Difficulties:	158
Unresolved Issues From Your Own Childhood:	160
Scapegoating:	161
The Anger-guilt-reparation Cycle:	162
Not Using The Strategies For All Of Your Children:	163
Hostility Towards Your Child:	164
Inadvertently supporting the creation of a 'Safe Zone':	165
Fear Of Change:	165
Lack of Support:	166
Lack Of Time:	166
Unresolved Trauma:	167
Coming Off Medication:	168
The Structure Of The Next Chapters:	171
Chapter 8 *Stress and assertiveness*	*172*
Dealing With Stress:	174
Being Assertive And Authoritative:	180
Relationship Patterns:	181
Chapter 9 *Separating the Child from the Problem*	*184*
Who Is Mr Temper And What Is He Like?	186
Chapter 10 *Consequences*	*188*
Primary School Aged Children:	191
Secondary School Children/ Teenagers:	195
Chapter 11 *Lifestyle and Family Life*	*201*
Changing Your Family Lifestyle:	202
Dietary Intervention:	203
Family Time:	210
Fresh Air And Exercise:	212
Television And Computer Games:	212

    Bedtime Routines: 213

    Responsibility, Trust and Independence: 217

    Support: 217

Chapter 12 *Working with schools*   *220*

    Improving The Learning Environment At Home: 222

    Get The Right Assessment And Help: 222

    Working With School To Close The Home/school Loop: 223

    Teaching Your Child Social Skills: 225

    If Necessary Change Schools: 228

Chapter 13 *Helping others with your Expertise*   *229*

    Building a First Aid Kit: 229

    Helping Others With Your Expertise: 229

Notes   **231**

About the Author   **239**

PREFACE

Early in the nineteenth century a new 'science' came into existence called 'Phrenology'. Phrenologists believed that by examining the shape and unevenness of a head or skull, you could discover facts about a person's intelligence and character traits. They thought that the brain was the location of the mind and that the brain is composed of distinct areas (which they called 'organs') each of which had a different function (for example an 'organ' for intelligence). They believed that the size of an 'organ' was a measure of its power. Finally they thought that the shape of the brain is determined by the development of these various brain 'organs' and that the skull takes its shape from the brain. Therefore they thought that by measuring the surface of the skull, you could get an accurate picture of a person's psychological abilities and tendencies.

Most phrenologists would run their bare fingertips over a head to distinguish any elevations or indentations. Sometimes callipers, measuring tapes and other instruments were used. A skilled phrenologist knew not just the layout of the head according to the latest phrenological chart, but also the personality traits associated with each of the 35 odd 'organs' (the number of brain 'organs' gradually increased over time). Like so many popular sciences, the phrenologists were only interested in evidence that confirmed their ideas. Phrenologists spent considerable time and effort defending themselves and their 'science' from criticism- always ready to portray themselves as Galileo-like defenders of natural 'truth'. Any evidence or anecdote which seemed to confirm that their 'science' was accurate, was promoted by them as 'proof' of the 'truth' of phrenology. What phrenologists never accepted was that a psychological characteristic could be independent of the size of its 'organ'.

Phrenology Societies were established and 'scientific' journals were developed. At the dawn of the twentieth century nearly a hundred years after phrenology was first described, phrenologists were still attracting mass audiences to their lectures and 'skull reading' sessions. Phrenologists' campaigned for their beliefs, that the protuberances on the skull provided an accurate index of talents and abilities, to be applied to education and criminal reform and they suggested that phrenology could be used to determine the most suitable career for the young.

Phrenology, as all popular fads, eventually became unfashionable, gradually degenerated into a sect of zealous extremists, and the practice slowly disappeared. Nevertheless, the British Phrenological Society (founded in 1887) was only disbanded in 1967. A legacy of phrenology lived on in other projects of measuring and comparing human heads- most notoriously the attention given to cranial size and forehead shape (which houses the frontal lobe) which was used by late 19th and early 20th century racial anthropologists (and later Nazi anthropologists) to confirm their belief that Europeans were superior to other humans (interestingly, with ADHD a small frontal lobe is again being suggested as the cause of immature behaviour).

In its heyday phrenology was seen as a robust science that measured 'real' qualities in people- in other words a science that could tell you some 'truth' about the person under study. What is not surprising when poor science comes to be seen as factual beyond dispute is that its conclusions sat comfortably with the social values and beliefs of the society within which it developed. Thus phrenologists' claim that their science 'proved' that non-Europeans had lower intelligence found support in the racist beliefs of the time, that perpetuated the idea that their Empires reflected a 'natural' hierarchy. If phrenology's conclusions were in opposition to that of the society, it is unlikely that an idea with such a slim scientific basis would have lasted as long as it did.

Many professionals and academics, including myself, are concerned that we are today witnessing the creation of a 'new phrenology'. In the last couple of decades many inventions have given us a new window on the brain. We have computers that can generate a three dimensional picture of x-rays of a person's brain, allowing us to measure the size of different structures and different parts of the brain. We have totally new kinds of brain imaging devices that allow us to see the brain in action. Thus we can measure blood flow to different parts of the brain, or see which parts of the brain are using more energy whilst someone is doing an activity (like trying to solve a puzzle). This type of scan is called 'functional neuroimaging' because it gives you information about the brain whilst the brain is doing something (functioning).

These new brain scans have caused much excitement in the psychiatric community and researchers have set about measuring the brains, and its internal structures, in people with a variety of psychiatric diagnoses, in an attempt to find evidence of differences in these people's brains compared to the rest of the population. No markers in the brain have been found for any of the psychiatric diagnoses studied. Despite this disappointing failure, it has not stopped some academics making wildly exaggerated claims about these brain-scanning studies. One such area is ADHD (see chapters1 and 2).

The problem when professionals and academics make conclusions not supported by the scientific evidence and further insists that their conclusions are the truth and only truth is that you end up in similar situation to that of the (so-called) science of phrenology. If the conclusions fit with the beliefs and interests of those in powerful positions in society, then the question of the strength of the scientific evidence can be overlooked. All that is needed is for a group of high status individuals to say that their pet theory is not simply an idea, it is a 'scientific fact', and the path for this idea to become viewed as 'scientific fact' is cleared. Furthermore, in the absence of objective methods to verify these theories (such as a medical test) there is an ever-present danger that such speculative concepts like ADHD will be misused by those in a position of power to perpetuate social inequality and as justification for oppressing the powerless (as happened with phrenology).

ADHD has come to be viewed as an inherited disease of the brain long before any evidence to show this had been found. Brain scan studies then set out to find the evidence to back up this theory. Even though these brain scan studies have not produced reliable, proven and reproducible results that demonstrate some consistent abnormality can be found in the brains of children diagnosed with ADHD (see chapters 1and 2), it has not stopped the big players in the field (like the phrenologists of old) saying that the evidence is indisputable.

The new phrenologists like the phrenologists of old are having great difficulty defending the scientific basis of their beliefs. Like the phrenologists of old they are afraid of an open debate and instead use their current position of power to demonise opposition and paint themselves as Galileo-like defenders of natural 'truth'. Thus in 2002 a group of prominent pro-ADHD academics and clinicians produced an *'International Consensus Statement on ADHD'*. The authors start by saying *"We, the undersigned consortium of international scientists, are deeply concerned about the periodic inaccurate portrayal of attention deficit hyperactivity disorder (ADHD) in media reports. This is a disorder with which we are all very familiar and toward which many of us have dedicated scientific studies if not entire careers. We fear that inaccurate stories rendering ADHD as myth, fraud, or benign condition may cause thousands of sufferers not to seek treatment for their disorder. It also leaves the public with a general sense that this disorder is not valid or real or consists of a rather trivial affliction"*, and finish with *"To publish stories that ADHD is a fictitious disorder or merely a conflict between today's Huckleberry Finns and their caregivers is tantamount to declaring the earth flat, the laws of gravity debatable, and the periodic table in chemistry a fraud. ADHD should be depicted in the media as realistically and accurately as it is depicted in science—as a valid disorder having varied and substantial adverse impact on those who may suffer from it through no fault of their own or their parents and teachers"*.

There are many cultural and political reasons why the idea that there is such a thing as ADHD caused by an abnormality in children's brains became popular in Western society. There have been changes in the way we view childhood, child rearing and education which all contribute to changing ideas about what a normal child should be like (see chapters 2, 3 and 4). These changes have particularly affected our view of boys (who are 3 to 10 times more likely to be diagnosed with ADHD than girls). Perhaps one of the most worrying is the idea that ADHD is an inherited brain abnormality. This has opened the floodgates for using largely untested and potentially addictive psychiatric drugs on children whose developing brains may be highly vulnerable to their side effects. This meant the second most powerful industry in the world (after the arms industry) could now pour its resources into promoting this idea with many consequent knock-on effects which I discuss in the first half of the book.

So, as you may have gathered this book takes a sceptical look at the whole phenomena of ADHD, its diagnosis and its treatment. I have written this book to try and reach out to parents who are struggling with trying to understand what this thing called ADHD is all about, what relevance it has to their children, and what they can do to help their children if they are concerned about them having ADHD. I have divided the book into two halves. The first half deals with theory and the second half is a practical guide to things that you can do to help your children without needing to turn to medication. Although the temptation may be to completely skip the first half and go straight to the second half I urge you not to do this. In fact, if you were just going to read one half of the book I would suggest you read the first half. This in itself may prove help enough to change your thinking about and your understanding of ADHD, which may be enough to lead you to have sufficient acceptance of the types of problems you have with your children to not want to do anything more active about it. Often it is just this change in perspective and enhanced understanding that can be enough.

One of the fears for many parents when I tell them I do not believe that ADHD is a medical condition, is that they become concerned that I am therefore blaming them for their child's problems, see them as bad parents and that it is bad parenting that is causing the problems. Whilst I am not shy in explaining to parents things that I think they need to do differently, I am very clear that it is extremely rare for me to see, what I would consider to be a bad parent in my clinical practice. On the whole 'bad parents' are those who are neglecting their children on *purpose*, and even then there are often some very sad and unfortunate circumstances that these 'neglectful' parents are struggling with.

In my opinion, parent blaming and child blaming (which I consider diagnoses such as ADHD to be doing) are opposites sides of the same coin. As I hope you will discover through reading this book, both parents and, in particular, children are vulnerable to becoming the targets to blame for all sorts of other failures in our cultures (such as failures of the school system, government policies, and workplace practices). What I do think is useful to bear in mind, however, is that not blaming the parent or the children does not mean that parents and children should not take responsibility for their behaviour. Many of the suggestions in the second half are about helping you and your children through that process of gaining and taking responsibility for the way you behave as one way to begin to free yourselves and your children from the oppressive messages and practices that so many families have to cope with in the modern world.

Acknowledgements

Thanks to my wonderful wife and three children: Michelle, Lewis and Zoe, for their love, patience and support and for teaching me so much. Thanks to all the rest of my family and friends who 'have been there' when we have gone through difficult times. Thanks to my current employers Lincolnshire Partnership NHS Trust, for allowing me the time and freedom to write (though I should note that the views mentioned in this book are my own and do not necessarily represent the views of my employers). Thanks to my wife Kitty, for her help in typing, preparing and commenting on the text. Thanks to my colleagues and staff at Ash Villa, the Spalding and Holbeach, the Scunthorpe, and the Grimsby, Community Child and Adolescent Mental Health Teams, for their reflection, comments and critiques of my ideas and practice. Thanks to all the other colleagues I correspond and carry out academic endeavours with, who have helped me learn so much, in particular (in no particular order) Begum Maitra, Jonathan Leo, Carl Cohen, Brad Lewis, Kenneth Thompson, Ann Miller, Brian McCabe, Neil Gardner, Joanna Moncrieff, Phil Thomas, Pat Bracken, Duncan Double, Eia Asen, Basant Puri, Janice Hill, Steve Carver-Smith, Bob Johnston, Jacky Scott-Coombes, Katy Brown, Mandy Brown, and Samuel Ted-Aggrey. Thanks to Natalie Glynn my publishing advisor at Author House. Finally, Thanks to Palgrave MacMillan for permission to re-publish some of the arguments I first used in *Naughty Boys*, my 2005 book published with them.

PART 1

THEORETICAL PERSPECTIVES

Chapter 1

Myths and facts

In this chapter I tackle head-on some of the claims made by those who believe ADHD is a diagnosis that indicates something is wrong in the brain of the child/person with the diagnosis. I hope you can read this with an open mind and please be clear that I am not saying that there isn't a problem, or that difficult and stigmatising behaviours don't exist that can understandably attract the label ADHD. Please also understand that I am not blaming the parent or for that matter the child. Years of clinical experience (and years as a parent myself) has made me appreciate just how hard life can be, what obstacles parents face in today's world, and how confusing it can become when different professionals tell you different things. It is very rare indeed for me to see parents who have negative intentions toward their children, it is the good parents who wish to seek help for their children and it takes much noble humility to decide to seek help and face having to make some changes. What I am trying to do in this chapter is simply to get you to ask some questions about the idea that ADHD is a biologically based brain disorder and that we know how to work out who has this brain problem from who doesn't.

Myth 1: Attention deficit hyperactivity disorder (ADHD) is a mental illness/psychiatric disorder that can be reliably diagnosed and occurs in similar numbers of children regardless of their cultural background. It affects between 3 and 10% percent of all children, is a lifelong disorder and leads to serious disability in the young person's ability to learn, socialise, work, and otherwise lead a normal life.

Facts and discussion: There are no medical tests for ADHD. There are no specific brain functioning tests for ADHD. There are no specific psychological tests for ADHD. There are no specific observational tests for ADHD. A doctor, through that doctor's assessment of a child's history and reported behaviour problems, makes a diagnosis of ADHD. Rating scales, which the child's parents or carers and teachers fill out about the child concerned, are frequently used to assist the doctor when they are assessing a child for ADHD. These rating scales are questionnaires in which adults looking after the child (most usually a separate questionnaire for a parent/carer and a separate questionnaire for a teacher) are asked to decide on the frequency with which hyperactive, inattentive, or impulsive behaviours are occurring in the child. They are not a test for ADHD as all a rating questionnaire can measure is an adult's opinion about a particular child's behaviour at a particular moment in time and in a particular setting.

Common questions used in rating scales (which the person filling in the questionnaire has to rate for frequency or severity in the child) include[1]:

- Often fails to give close attention to details or makes careless mistakes in homework, work, or other activities.

- Often has difficulties sustaining attention in tasks or play activities.

- Often does not seem to listen when spoken to directly.

- Often does not follow through instructions and fails to finish schoolwork, chores, or duties in the workplace.

- Often has difficulties organizing tasks and activities.

- Often avoids, dislikes or is reluctant to engage in tasks that require sustained mental efforts.

- Often loses things necessary for tasks or activities (e.g. toys, school assignments, pencils, books).

- Is often easily distracted by extraneous stimuli.

- Is often forgetful in daily activities.

- Often fidgets with hands or feet or squirms in seat.

- Often leaves seat in classroom or in other situations in which remaining seated is expected.

- Often runs about or climbs excessively in situations in which it is inappropriate.

- Often has difficulty playing or engaging in leisure activities quietly.

- Is often "on the go" or often acts as if "driven by a motor".

- Often talks excessively.

- Often blurts out answers before questions have been completed.
- Often has difficulty waiting their turn.
- Often interrupt or intrudes on others.

As you can see words such as 'often', 'seems', 'difficulties', 'reluctant', 'easily', 'quietly', and 'excessively' that appear in these questionnaires are hard to define. For example the word 'often' appears in every one of the above questions, but what does it mean? Does it mean that the child does those behaviours at least once a day or at least once a minute? These questionnaires can only rate a particular adult's perception of a particular child at a particular moment in time and in a particular setting. In other words they are measures of the *subjective* perception of the adult filling in the rating scale. What they cannot be is an *objective* factual piece of 'hard data' that measures something intrinsic to the child.

These days when making a diagnosis of ADHD, the doctor doing the evaluation does not need to observe the behaviours of hyperactivity, impulsivity, or inattention in the child concerned during the assessment. Making the diagnosis is based on taking a history (to see if the behaviours, according to those giving the doctor the history, started early in a child's life, and to exclude any other medical reason that may be causing the behavioural problems) and evaluating a couple of rating questionnaires. It's not what you might call 'rocket science', and ultimately the making of the diagnosis (or not) rests on the beliefs of the doctor and how they interpret the history and questionnaires. It's an entirely subjective process.

Hyperactivity, impulsivity and poor concentration are behaviours that occur on a continuum. All children, particularly boys, will present with such behaviour in some settings at some point. I know this as a parent myself. They are not behaviours that would be interpreted as abnormal whenever they occur. Contrast this to a hallucination (such as hearing voices that are not there) or a delusion which, in Western culture at least, are viewed as abnormal in most circumstances (However, even with these symptoms that are psychiatrically categorised as 'psychotic' symptoms- in other words symptoms of someone deemed to be out of touch with reality- it is not as straight forward as many believe. For example, it is now recognized that many otherwise healthy and socially well functioning people sometimes hear voices).

Without any medical tests to establish which individual has a physical problem causing these behaviour problems, defining the cut off between normal and ADHD is arrived at by an arbitrary decision. Those who have argued that ADHD does not exist as a real disorder, often start by pointing this out. Because of this uncertainty about definition it is hardly surprising that epidemiological studies (studies that measure how many have a disorder) have produced very different prevalence rates for ADHD ranging from about 0.5% of school age children to 26% of school age children[2].

ADHD studies have found three to five times more boys than girls qualify for the diagnosis (and something like five to ten times more boys than girls get prescribed medication for ADHD). This is very similar to the gender distribution found more generally in psychiatric disorders during the pre-adolescent years. This is mostly made up of 'behavioural disorders' like ADHD, Conduct Disorder, and Oppositional Defiant Disorder. Why is it that the behaviour of boys is seen as a particular problem during the primary school years? This seemingly obvious question is rarely discussed in the psychiatric academic literature (though extensively in other academic circles such as sociology, anthropology and cultural studies).

What sort of brain problem are we attempting to categorise here? Is it that boys generally have bad genes compared to girls? Is it something to do with the normal biological differences between male and female genes? Is there an interaction between boy's behaviour and changes in social expectations regarding children's behaviour generally? Do social changes in family structure, lifestyles, teaching methods, classroom sizes, rates of violence, rates of substance misuse and so on have an effect on our perceptions and beliefs about boy's and girl's behaviour, or on their behaviour directly? Has life got harder for boys in some way? Has life got harder for parents trying to control normal boy behaviour? Are we still compelled to pay more attention to the behaviour of boys than that of girls, only now we medicalise this (studies show that adults in Western societies are usually more tolerant of hyperactivity in girls than in boys)[3]? Do changes in teaching methods and a predominance of female teachers have an effect on how we understand and deal with boys' behaviour? These and other social/cultural questions relating to ADHD are rarely discussed in the medical literature (although I do discuss them at length in my book *Naughty Boys: Anti-Social Behaviour, ADHD and the Role of Culture*).

If ratings of hyperactivity, poor concentration and disruptiveness are subjective then it is likely that we will find large differences in the way these behaviours are viewed in different cultures. This is indeed what is found. One finding from many studies, for example, is an apparently high rate of ADHD in children from China and Hong Kong. In these studies nearly three times as many Chinese as English children were rated as 'hyperactive'. However, when the researchers came to examine the results more closely they found that it was Chinese doctors rating Chinese children as hyperactive and that these 'hyperactive' Chinese children would not have been rated as hyperactive by most English doctors. In fact they turned out to be a good deal less hyperactive than English children rated as 'hyperactive'[4]. One suggestion for this finding is that it may be due to the great importance of school success in Chinese culture leading to an intolerance of much lesser degrees of disruptive behaviour. Whatever the reasons, it demonstrates that hyperactivity and disruptiveness is highly dependent on how your culture interprets the significance of such behaviour. This is further confirmed when you look at clinical practice within a country, let alone between them. For example, studies have found that the rate of diagnosis of ADHD varied by a factor of ten from county to county within the same state (in the United States)[5].

Many cultures simply do not see the behaviours we label as ADHD as being a problem. For example in a study carried out in a middle class, Mexican school (whose teachers and local doctors knew about ADHD), using standard rating questionnaires the researchers found that about 8% of the children could be diagnosed as having ADHD, yet there was only one child in that school (of over 200 pupils) with the diagnosis. Through interviews with parents and teachers the researchers found that they regarded ADHD-type behaviours as normal for those children's ages[6].

There is also a more complicated issue that we need to be aware of in any discussion about the where to place the boundary when diagnosing ADHD. This relates to the concept of 'co-morbidity'. When psychiatrists talk about 'co-morbidity' they mean that more than one diagnosis can be given to any particular patient. In other words a child diagnosed with ADHD may also have symptoms that mean they can be given another psychiatric diagnosis, for example an 'anxiety disorder'. In such a case this child would be said to have ADHD with 'co-morbid' anxiety disorder (or visa versa- an anxiety disorder with co-morbid ADHD). Numerous studies demonstrate the high frequency with which these supposedly separate child psychiatric disorders occur in individuals with ADHD. It is estimated that about half the children with ADHD also have a conduct disorder, about half also have an emotional disorder, about one third have an anxiety disorder and another third have major depression. Co-morbidity is so widespread that *at least* three quarters of ADHD diagnosed children will have at least one other diagnosable child psychiatric condition. What does this all mean?

Psychiatrists use co-morbidity as a way of trying to explain clinical reality when it does not appear to match the diagnostic categories that researchers use. It's a way of maintaining a fantasy that there is a natural, probably biological, boundary between psychiatric disorders, where no natural boundaries exist. Thus we have another problem of how to interpret the meaning of the evidence in ADHD. How many of the studies that we have on ADHD are actually telling us more about a co-morbid disorder than ADHD? How relevant to clinical practice are studies that have ruled out co-morbidity before studying the affected individuals, given that most children with ADHD that professionals like myself see in clinics, will have at least one other co-morbid disorder? How relevant are guidelines on treating ADHD when little research is being done on such treatment's effects on co-morbid disorders? But perhaps most importantly does the high rate of co-morbidity suggest that ADHD is more useful as a concept to researchers than to clinicians, as in real life situations straightforward, uncomplicated ADHD is rare? If this is the case then our current knowledge base on ADHD is close to useless (castles built on sand), and current practice (which rarely acknowledges co-morbidity, and when it does so seems unable to step back and see the 'big picture' and instead focuses on each diagnosis as if they are separate features of the child) seriously misguided.

Because of these serious problems about how to define ADHD, it is hard to know what to make of follow-up studies. For example some studies that show a higher number of young people with ADHD have accidents when they are compared to those who don't have ADHD. This is, in scientific terms is known as an association; you cannot say that ADHD causes the sufferer to have more accidents as another factor could explain both. For example is it that the study has simply found that more boys have accidents than girls, or that it was a co-morbid condition (like conduct disorder) that is more responsible, or a totally unrelated factor responsible for both causing ADHD and accidents (such as learning difficulties, low self-esteem, stress in the family, poor diet etc.). We could also get stuck in a circular argument about ADHD as you might then decide to define ADHD at the point where there is enough of a percentage increase in accidents over the rest of children and then use that as your evidence that ADHD exists as a 'real' thing.

From a philosophical point of view this lack of objective tests, confusion on how define the cut-off point between normal and ADHD, cross-cultural differences, and high co-morbidity leaves the practice of diagnosing ADHD stuck in a philosophical whirlpool that goes something like this: What is causing this child's hyperactivity and poor concentration? Answer: ADHD. How do you know it's ADHD? Answer: because they have poor concentration and are hyperactive. Of course you can say the same thing about all the other co-morbid diagnosis (like Oppositional Defiant Disorder, conduct disorder and so on). It really is based on astonishingly sloppy and unscientific thinking.

To really confuse matters there is a long list of famous scientists (like Albert Einstein and Isaac Newton), authors (like Hans Christian Anderson and Lewis Carroll), inventors (like Thomas Edison and Michael Faraday), artists (like Leonardo da Vinci and Salvador Dali), politicians (like Winston Churchill and Abraham Lincoln), actors (like Sylvester Stallone and Steve McQueen), musicians (like Beethoven and Ozzy Osbourne), sportsmen (like Michael Jordan and Paul Gascoigne) and comedians (like Billy Connolly and Jim Carrey) all said to have had (or have) ADHD. The list is endless[7]. What does this mean? What sort of a 'disorder' is this if it is associated with such 'greatness'? If it is ADHD that has driven these people to 'think outside the box' and end up contributing so much to our culture, would 'treating' ADHD deprive us of the creativity and inspiration that such people bring, and send us, as a culture into some sort of dull, homogenous middle ground? For many of the above famous names, their main issue as children was surviving the school system where they attracted labels like stupid, lazy and un-teachable. If the problem here is not these individuals' innate abilities, but a mismatch between them and their schools, is it the kids or their schooling environments that we should be changing?

Myth 2: ADHD is caused by irregularities in brain chemistry and runs in families. Scientists have identified malfunctioning genes that disrupt communications between different cells in parts of the brain that are in charge of self-control and inhibition. Scientists have demonstrated an abnormality in the brains of children with ADHD.

Fact and discussion: No other child psychiatric disorder has received more attention in biological research than ADHD. There are over thirty brain scan studies of children diagnosed with ADHD that have occurred over the past three decades. Taken together these studies have not uncovered a consistent abnormality and have suggested a wide variety of different brain structures as being involved. In none of these brain scan studies have the brains of the children diagnosed with ADHD been considered in any way clinically abnormal.

The most widely debated issue is whether any of the minor differences these studies have found between the brains of children diagnosed with ADHD and the normal controls, were due to the medication most of the children diagnosed with ADHD in the studies were taking. After all, animal studies have found that that taking stimulants can cause a long lasting change in the brain biochemistry of rats. The one scientific way to address this question is for a study to be carried out where children who have never been exposed to medication and who are diagnosed with ADHD are compared to an age matched control group.

In 2002 a group of researchers published a study that claimed to have done this. This study included three groups: 49 children diagnosed with ADHD that had never received medication, 103 ADHD children who had received medication (although no information was given as to how much and for how long) and 139 'normal' children who made up the 'control group'. Thus the authors had an opportunity to make numerous comparisons between the three groups the most important being between the unmedicated group and the control group. However, compared to the control group, the unmedicated ADHD group were two years younger, and were shorter and lighter. This meant that all the researchers managed to demonstrate in their comparison was that older children had bigger brains than younger ones! What the authors chose to highlight instead was that there was no significant difference between the brain sizes of the unmedicated group and the medicated group and this was then used to conclude that medication is not causing the difference found in the brain scanning studies.

This is fraught with problems, particularly as they provide no detailed information with regards the medication profile of the medicated group. It remains the case that the simplest way to settle the argument is to compare the brains of an unmedicated group with an age matched control group, which was not done in this study. Interestingly, given the size of the control group it is still feasible for the authors to do this with their existing sample and they have been challenged to do just that (choose a more age matched control group from a sub-sample of their existing control group and compare these to the unmedicated group), but thus far they have not done this. One has to wonder why[8].